Sunny Side Up
Health and Happiness by the Dozen

Cheryl B. Fell, RN-BC
"Nurse FUNshine"

www.SunnySideUpBook.com

Timmy,

It's great [to see?] you happy and [...] life. See you in March.

Cheryl
4/28/13

Nurse FUNshine

Sunny Side Up: Health and Happiness by the Dozen

Copyright © 2011 Cheryl B. Fell. All rights reserved. No part of this book may be reproduced or retransmitted in any form or by any means without the written permission of the publisher.

Published by Wheatmark®
610 East Delano Street, Suite 104, Tucson, Arizona 85705 U.S.A.
www.wheatmark.com

ISBN: 978-1-60494-502-7
LCCN: 2010932167

This book is dedicated in loving memory to my Granny Mitchell, who lived to be 102. Granny's sunny disposition, quick wit and competitive spirit made her a joy to be around. Granny's unconditional love and homemade goodies always made me feel special on the inside. Thank you Granny Mitchell for being my treasured example of health and happiness and teaching me how to live sunny side up.

Contents

Page 1   *Chapter 1*
              **Breakfast of Champions ...
              Eggcelent Choice**

Page 11   *Chapter 2*
              **All Scrambled Up and
              Going No Where**

Page 21   *Chapter 3*
              **Who Cares Whether the
              Chicken or the Egg Came
              First? I Want to Act Like a
              Goose!**

Page 25   *Chapter 4*
              Confrontation Over Easy

Page 27	*Chapter 5* **Hard Boiled Boundaries**
Page 31	*Chapter 6* **Eggstra Ha-Ha-Ho-Ho-He-He**
Page 38	*Chapter 7* **Don't Be a Chicken!**
Page 45	*Chapter 8* **A "Free-Range" Home**
Page 50	*Chapter 9* **Baby Chicks ... Tickle Them, Please!**
Page 59	*Chapter 10* **Cracking Up**
Page 66	*Chapter 11* **Empty Nesters ... YES!**
Page 70	*Chapter 12* **Roosters Rule the World with Wisdom**
Page 75	*Baker's Dozen* **Living on the Sunny Side of the Street**

1

Breakfast of Champions ... Eggcelent Choice

*Wake up and smell the coffee! It's
time to face the daily grind.
Hurry, hurry don't be late, and remember to be kind.*

*Another hectic schedule overflows my cup.
Is it really Monday? Who's going to walk the pup?*

*Why can't we sleep in late and
leisurely sip coffee in our bed?
The alarm goes off for the second
time ... oh my aching head.*

*Today's triple shot espresso better
jump-start my morning routine.
See you later alligator; I'll be home at 6:15.*

*No time for breakfast what a shame, the
most important meal of the day.
I guess I'll run on empty and will
myself through another day.*

*Traffic here, traffic there, morning traffic everywhere.
Uptight drivers in a world of their
own, does anyone really care?*

*Something's got to give I say,
how can we live this fast?
A little voice whispers in my ear ...
"Remember the ways of your past."*

One day as I was driving to work on I-10 in crazy Baton Rouge traffic, I composed this poem and thought about the "good old days" of my childhood at Grandma's house. I reminisced about Granny's breakfasts and what made them healthy meals. Fresh squeezed orange juice, whole grain toast, and endless eggs of course. Poached eggs, fried eggs, soft boiled eggs, scrambled eggs, eggs in a basket, omelets, french toast, waffles, and pancakes. Growing up I thought it was the eggs that made breakfast of champions. "Looking back, I realize that gathering at Granny's table for breakfast made my cousins, sisters, brother and me feel special. We shared our dreams and goals with each other and Granny's unconditional acceptance made us feel like real champions, ready to conquer the day." Grandma started a Breakfast Club with her very own grandchildren and she didn't even know it! Granny's Breakfast Club changed us from the inside out and we learned how to live sunny side up. Yes indeed, the **"C"** word was present at our Breakfast Club. Breakfast of Champions Part I at Granny's planted seeds of health and happiness deep within our souls. We changed and grew up and life went on.

One morning in my early 30s I woke up sick and tired of being sick and tired. My adult girlfriends and I gathered for breakfast while our children were at school. Our conversation began as small talk, then we got honest about our pursuit toward happiness. We all agreed that we were merely existing day after day instead of really living life. The four of us made a conscious decision to seek positive change in our lives. Something powerful happened that morning at our Breakfast Club when we humbly surrendered and accepted the fact that inner soul work was required if we wanted to transform our lives from ordinary to extra ordinary.

We vowed to change, but this time, it would be everlasting change. Everyone laughed. We remembered our repeated attempts to change. We had tried exercise plans, competitive sports, fad diets, meditation, new wardrobes, retreats, counseling, vacations, new jobs, bigger houses, fancy cars, personal trainers, life coaches, how-to books, and various hobbies only to discover that health and happiness didn't last. There is no "quick fix" for living sunny side up. Wellness is a way of life.

My girlfriends and I agreed that awareness and willingness were the first steps towards authentic change. Starting that very day, when we did the same things over and over, we would notice our thoughts, attitudes and behaviors. For the first time, we embraced the truth that we needed to change our perceptions in order to change our lives. Perhaps our own resistance to change had been our biggest obstacle.

We agreed to meet again the next day for Breakfast of Champions Part II and share the outcome of our awareness experiment. We would openly and honestly explore how mindfulness affected our emotional well-being and daily spiritual path. Everyone giggled with skepticism; yet we were all willing to take on the challenge to change.

Below are some useful tips that helped our Breakfast Club cope with change. Perhaps you can start with one or two strategies, then repeat the behaviors until they occur naturally. Once you accomplish one or two positive changes, set additional goals and implement a few more suggestions.

Eggcelent Goals Change Us from the Inside Out

- Know that change will require you to think and act outside your "safe" daily routines

- Jump-start your attitude every morning with gratitude
- Be excited about your potential and the future
- Expect progress, not perfection
- Establish reasonable, attainable and measurable goals
- Focus on your goals instead of your struggles
- Acknowledge positive accomplishments no matter how small
- Use your time and energy towards fine tuning your own strengths and best qualities
- Evaluate progress on a regular basis
- Take time to celebrate and reward success
- Learn to take yourself "lightly" and your life seriously
- Discover, develop and kindle your sense of humor
- Let go of the past. Forgiveness equals freedom
- Move beyond anger, shame, fear and guilt
- Remain flexible so you won't get "bent out of shape"
- Choose not to participate in gossip
- Listen with your heart, not just your ears
- Practice responding instead of reacting
- Learn to love your job or seek a career that fuels your passion
- Become your own best friend
- Think positive thoughts before going to sleep each night
- Communicate with God. Pray for wisdom, courage and strength, essential elements to sustain everlasting change.

Day 2 began our journey towards the pursuit of health and happiness. Our Breakfast Club began precisely at 6:00 am. We all agreed that timeliness was an essential factor in becoming a happy and serene individual. Besides, our busy schedules allowed only 30 minutes for our gathering. A nutritious breakfast was served and the conversation took off.

One by one we shared our observations, thoughts and behaviors from the previous day. Some reviewed journal entries while some went over lists. Some looked in their daily planner; some read notes from little pieces of paper, and some depended on their memory. Everyone's approach to change was different, yet we all had the common denominator of desire followed by accountability. One by one, we each made a commitment to this group of champions and the pursuit of health and happiness. We would encourage, care, cheer, confront, challenge and congratulate one another for the sake of positive change. Plus five days a week, we would receive a delicious home cooked breakfast. Eggcelent choice!

After breakfast, Day 2 consisted of a whole lot of noticing, biting our tongues, stopping negative thoughts from messing with our optimism and differentiating between our own biased perceptions vs. reality.

After one long day of this so-called heightened awareness, we came to the breakfast table on Day 2 tired, but we had acquired valuable knowledge about accepting life on life's terms. We agreed to set realistic short-term goals that would eventually lead to satisfying long-term goals and ultimate happiness. Our goals included specific action steps that would help us achieve worthwhile change and happiness. "Real" change requires practice and hard work, but the freedom of joyful living is worth the blood, sweat and tears. We are the champions of the world!

Sharing was the number one priority on Day 3. Food became secondary. I know it's hard to believe we chose listening and sharing over eggs, but this noticing, wondering and reflecting over the past couple of days had left us feeling lighter. Perhaps it was because we came to the amazing conclusion that most of the stuff we thought about didn't really matter in the grand scheme of life.

Worrying doesn't get us anywhere. Fear paralyzes us. Being judgmental and critical drains our energy. The more we think positive and act like champions, the more we incorporate desirable behaviors into our everyday life. Being right was no longer our main focus. We wanted to be happy and free. Instead of being bitter, we strove to be better. Day 3 of our Breakfast Club was over at 6:30 am and the sun was shining. It was time to go out and practice our sunny side up techniques.

Day 4 and the breakfast of champions seemed like a team. In less than one week, we had come together as a powerful, life-changing group. Funny thing … no one felt the need to be the leader, yet each one of us brought something unique to the table. The respect among us felt awesome. Confidentiality was a given. Everyone was on time and anxious to share their progress or lack of progress.

It appeared that some team members did not have to apologize as much. They were processing words at a deeper level and this conscious decision-making helped them to respond instead of react. Others were still repeating some of their bad habits, but they reported the ability to "catch" their negative behaviors sooner which meant fewer apologies and less frustration. Some were realizing that life's lessons had to be learned over and over again until they were brought to their knees or lifted to a higher level of awareness.

Soul work was both challenging and rewarding. This newly acquired wisdom made everyone feel proud. Once we got to the sunny side of the street, there was no going back. Good stuff was happening and the Breakfast Club members were changing day by day. Our family and friends were beginning to take notice. We clapped and cheered out loud for small personal and professional victories. Go team!

Day 5 of the breakfast of champions. We had made it through an entire work week with no absences or lame excuses. Everyone smiled and nodded with a sense of accomplishment as we greeted each other that morning. We were starting to become comfortable with eye contact and affirming one another. One by one we shared the goals we had accomplished during the week, the goals we needed to extend into week two, the goals we wanted to modify, and the goals we decided to eliminate. Everyone made progress, some more than others, but it didn't matter because we were all genuinely striving to live sunny side up.

As much as we enjoyed getting together, eating delicious breakfasts, sharing our success stories and owning our shortcomings, everyone agreed that our Breakfast Club needed to start meeting once a week. That way, we would have more time to practice change, as well as evaluate our ability to sustain authentic living without the daily support from our Breakfast Club.

Stay strong champions! See you next Wednesday at the same time on the sunny side of the street. Until then, remember that meaningful change will bring us closer towards health and happiness.

Take the Choice Challenge

In your quest to live on the sunny side of the street, here is a tool you can use to maintain a positive path towards wellness. Create some type of record using a journal, day planner, notebook, etc. For one week keep track of each time you experience positive or negative thoughts/feelings/emotions/behaviors. Here are a few examples:

POSITIVE	NEGATIVE
Amazement	Annoyance
Amusement	Aggravation
Aha Moment	Anger
Compliment	Complaint
Encouragement	Criticism
Excitement	Fear
Giggle	Gossip
Kindness	Guilt
Hopefulness	Hurt
Joy	Judgment

Laughter	Lies
Praise	Pride
Peace	Pessimism
Satisfaction	Shame
Serenity	Sarcasm
Talent	Trouble
Wisdom	Worry

Simply make a mark or write down the frame of mind you encounter throughout each day for 7 days. Please do not review your notes, total your score, or analyze the outcome until you have completed this challenge for one full week. After one week, count the total number of positive and negative emotions you experienced. Do you notice any patterns? Perhaps you identified some strengths and valuable character traits that need validation.

Can you identify specific areas needing improvement? What thoughts/emotions appear to be controlling your life? Could there be some deep hurt, pain, anger or guilt that surfaces and resurfaces as negative feelings? Could you, no, would you be willing to explore what really lies beneath your anger and hurt?

Becoming a champion isn't easy, but it will be worth the effort. "Real" change requires emotional honesty, hard work and practice. Happiness is an inside job. When you truthfully take the choice challenge, it can be used as a baseline tool to measure your progress towards positive change. After all, change is a matter of choice and we live by our eggcelent choices.

2

All Scrambled Up and Going No Where

WE HUMAN BEINGS are all scrambled up and going no where. We live in a world of fast food, fast talk, fast track, and fast living. My advice is to slow down. Hopefully old age or frail health will not be the factor that forces us to slow down and relax.

As the members of our Breakfast Club discovered the transformational power of belonging to a genuine group, clarity and insight helped us balance our lives. Our weekly Breakfast Club provided constructive feedback, gave us motivation, and held us accountable for our choices.

As a life changing group, we identified that managing stress was the next step to health and happiness. We believed we were ready to learn simple, practical stress management techniques and incorporate them into our daily lives. By reducing stress, we may just find that we can get more done in less time. Imagine that!

There are many great books and experts on stress management to help this scrambled up world of ours. When we get to the breaking point of being scrambled and beaten, we buy a self help book or attend a stress management seminar. We have such great intentions when we read a book or attend a workshop. Once we think we understand the method, we go out and try to do it perfectly, just like the experts said. We don't realize that sometimes we actually create more stress when we try to be perfect and do it "right" 100% of the time.

Success, failure, high hopes, discouragement…a roller coaster of emotions followed by the inevitable….quit and go back to what we know, our old way of rushing through life, our comfort zone, our adrenaline rush. We run from ourselves trying to suppress our inner anxiety and insecurities. For others the old way is scarcely existing day after day after day. Procrastination, denial, avoidance, worrying, barely hanging on. Our old behaviors all lead to STRESS. Go figure. Perhaps the stress in your life will lead you to a Breakfast Club for a taste of serenity, a shot of courage and eggcelent advice.

If we are going to effectively manage stress, we need to first figure out where the majority of our stress comes from. Is it our family? Friends? Job? Hobbies? Finances? Commitments? Community Activities? Ourselves? Could we be our own worst enemy? Maybe, just maybe, the pressure and unrealistic expectations we place upon ourselves is the major source of our stress. No wonder we are all scrambled up and going no where! It's hard to believe that we could be a major contributor to our own personal and professional stress.

Sometimes reality strikes like lightening, leaving us shocked and amazed. Other times clarity and insight sink in slowly like the setting sun. Either way stress becomes a major obstacle towards optimum health and happiness. Yes indeed, anxiety can rob us of our health and happiness. Stress ... what stress?

Set aside ten **uninterrupted** minutes and honestly answer the following questions. Put a T or F after each statement. Please answer the way you truly feel today, not the way you want to feel or the way you think you should feel, but answer how you currently deal with stress at the present time.

Short but Simple Stress Test (True or False)

1. People often come to me with their problems and ask for my advice. I frequently feel drained from the emotional demands of life and feeling responsible for others.
2. I frequently find that I am working harder and want the desired change more than the person seeking my advice.
3. I find myself saying "yes" when I really need to say "no."
4. I am irritable, edgy and resentful more than I am carefree, patient and cheerful.
5. It's been weeks since I did something I really love

to do. When I do "relax" and participate in a leisure activity, I feel guilty or lazy.
6. I can't remember the last time I had a hearty ha-ha-ha laugh.
7. Seems like I go through most days on automatic pilot, trying to do as much as possible in as little time as possible.
8. I multi task through life and yet my "to do" list never ends.
9. I fill in every waking hour of my daily calendar with appointments, activities, errands, etc. I have a habit of checking my watch and clock often.
10. I work harder than anyone else at my current job and am overly critical of the way others work.
11. Procrastination is a way of life for me. I spend much more time thinking about what I need to do instead of taking action and completing tasks.
12. I frequently experience physical symptoms that my health practitioner says are directly related to stress.
13. I find myself drinking alcohol and/or self medicating on a regular basis to help me deal with stress.

Total the number of **TRUE** responses that you answered. The more **TRUE** answers you have, the greater the stress in your life. It's that simple. Now go back and review your **TRUE** answers.

Try to make a connection between people, places and things. Do you recognize any patterns? Could the predominant link be YOU? Yes, believe it or not, we play a part in our own inner turmoil. The good news is that we have the ability to manage and eliminate some of the stress in our life.

Below are stress management tips that can help unscramble your world of chaos. Read the list, then decide which one(s) you want to put into action. Practice using these tips and skills until they become a natural part of your behavior. Add a new tip or skill each week or month depending on your progress and pace. As your stress decreases, you may notice increased clarity regarding your wants, needs, likes and dislikes. Increased clarity contributes to a balanced life which in turn generates health and happiness.

Our Breakfast Club met on Wednesday. Eggs, fresh strawberries and bagels were served along with plenty of conversation and stress management tips. Every member agreed that no one really likes scrambled eggs; we prefer eggs sunny side up!

Simple Stress Management Tips

- Do not take on any additional commitments until you have taken the "Short But Simple Stress Test" and identified what areas of your life need to change in order to decrease stress.
- When someone (other than your boss) asks you to do something, buy yourself some time for reflection. Tell him that you will get back with him in a few minutes, hours, tomorrow or next week with an answer. Then step back from the pressure, review

your calendar, and ask yourself if you **truly** want to take on this responsibility. If yes, then go for it! If no, simply tell the person that you will not be able to do it because your plate is full. Please do not tell him all the things you are currently doing. Simply thank him for asking and decline the opportunity. Period. The more you practice this time- buffer stress management tip, the happier you will be about your "yes" choices.

- Sleep and be well. The goal is to get enough deep sleep so you feel rested in the morning. Create a bedtime ritual and try to go to bed around the same time each night. Turn off the alarm clock and sleep in one day a week. Allow yourself to wake up naturally to your body's own rhythm. What a refreshing treat!
- Wake up twenty minutes earlier during the work week. Use this time for prayer, meditation, exercise, or free time. When things don't go as planned, you will have a little extra time to deal with the morning mishaps. Imagine how your days will flow when you arrive at work a few minutes early instead of rushing to be on time or being late!
- Protect your think time. Cherish peaceful moments so you can better deal with life's challenges. Plan time regularly for meditation, prayer and reflection. Commute to and from work quietly. Take a lunch break everyday to get away from your work space and change your mind on purpose. Contemplation

and pondering may reveal intuitive ways to work smarter not harder.
- Eat a hearty breakfast. Take a natural, yeast free, gluten free multi-vitamin/mineral supplement daily **with** food. Eliminate or reduce your caffeine, sugar and alcohol intake. Stay away from artificial sweeteners. Gather regularly at the breakfast and dinner table for food and fellowship.
- Treat your body right by eating a well balanced diet. Plan your main entrees for one week. Instead of last minute meal stress, you already know what you are preparing for supper (dinner) and can build your salad and vegetables around the main entrée. Include other family members in the meal planning. Shop only once a week and buy essentials for your main entrees along with fruits and vegetables that are on sale and in season. Take leftovers to work for lunch. You will be less tempted to eat fast food and save some money too! Besides, when you go out to lunch with co-workers for a special occasion, you will truly enjoy the meal and conversation without stressing out about spending money or calories.
- Pamper your body and soul. Temporarily disconnect from life in the fast lane. Take a warm, uninterrupted aromatherapy bath while listening to soothing music. Sit in a rocker or chair on your front porch and happily observe nature. Treat yourself to a massage or pedicure in a quiet spa setting.

- Notice and connect with your breathing during waking hours. Make a conscious habit of taking slow, deep breaths throughout the day. Deep breathing is beneficial when you feel tense or anxious. Breathe in through your nose and out through your mouth. As you exhale gently force the left over air out of your lungs. Try to get at least 10 minutes of fresh air daily.
- Engage in moderate exercise on a regular basis. Going on a brisk walk three or more times a week is an easy, free exercise. If you can still talk while you walk, your pace is about right.
- Loosen up your emotions. Avoid loneliness. Go to a movie with someone who loves to laugh and is not afraid to cry.
- Read a good book just for the fun of it. Reading a tear-jerker or humorous story can help release pent-up emotions.
- Simplify your life. Clean out your closets, files, and storage areas regularly. Sell, give away, or throw out anything you have not used in the past year. Organize your home and work space so you can find things. Put things away where they belong immediately after using them. Creating order out of chaos will help eliminate the fatiguing stress of losing things.
- Designate a drawer, closet, or cabinet for gifts. Stock up on gift certificates and presents for children and adults when you are shopping and have some extra money. Instead of rushing around to buy a gift at the last minute, you simply choose something from

your stash. All you have to do is wrap it. In addition, you may want to buy a greeting card file. Stock up on birthday cards, get well cards, wedding cards, sympathy cards, etc. The next time you need a card, all you have to do is go to your file and find the perfect card!

- "Lighten Up" the standards and pressures you put upon yourself so you can deal with the issues and tasks that are top priorities. The world won't end because the supper dishes are in the sink when you go to bed or the grass is a little longer than you like it.
- Don't expect everyone to be in a good mood or to like you. View annoying, aggravating people as teachers. Each of us is learning lessons on our journey through life. Perhaps that rude sales clerk is teaching us that respect is an essential component of customer service. Maybe the apathetic furniture warehouse employee is doing the best he can considering his personal battles day in and day out. Could we learn to be empathetic towards him and others? How about a lesson in gratitude for the obstacles we've overcome that contributed to our personal growth? The next time someone pushes your button, step back from the power struggle, smile and remember that even jerks can teach us something worthwhile about ourselves.
- Life is about waiting. Seems like we spend time each day waiting in line for something or someone. Why not make it a habit to plan for waiting and use this free time wisely? Have something readily available

in your car, purse, brief case, or laptop to work on while you wait. Perhaps you can read a book or magazine, pay some bills, send someone a greeting card, make your grocery list, review your daily planner for the next couple of days, or write in your journal. You will be amazed how fast the wait time goes and instead of being frustrated and uptight, you will feel good about accomplishing something productive.

- And last, but not least, put yourself on the top of your own "to do" list. One of the best stress management tips is learning how to take care of you first. When your own physical, emotional and spiritual needs are met, you will have the energy, joy and compassion to help others. You may still feel scrambled up occasionally, but for the most part you will be living over easy with your sunny side up.

3

Who Cares Whether the Chicken or the Egg Came First? I Want to Act Like a Goose!

WE'VE ALL HEARD the expression "silly goose," but actually, geese have many admirable qualities. Did you know that a flock of geese flies in a "V" formation? Do you know why? It's done because every member of the flock accepts the leadership role when needed. When the head goose becomes weary, a fresh goose from back in the pack flies forward and accepts the leadership position. Teamwork allows the flock to reorganize in order to maintain the fastest pace possible for the greatest good of the flock.

Another notable quality of geese is that they migrate

according to the weather. The reason for this is simple. They change their location and environment according to their needs. Geese would perish as a species if they were unable to adapt to changing conditions.

In addition, geese are fierce defenders. If you have ever crossed the path of a goose, you know what I'm talking about. There is something very intimidating about a hissing, honking goose that puffs up its feathers in an attempt to scare you away.

Our weekly Breakfast Club has become like a flock of geese. Together, we reinforce healthy change and look at life from a different point of view. Once upon a time we were chickens, but now we are a cohesive flock of geese. We are free to be ourselves. We are content flying together or alone. Sometimes we are leaders and other times we are followers. We discovered that transformation happens when we change our thinking and surrender our individual expectations for the good of the group. Acceptance, teamwork and willingness to change are major steps towards freedom.

Like geese, which fly ever forward and never look back, we now realize that we no longer want to be victims. We have quit blaming the world for our problems and unhappiness. We have accepted the fact that life isn't fair, our childhood could have been better, shit happens, the economy is in turmoil, and we really don't like other people telling us what to do.

The truth of the matter is that there is at least one thing we really don't like about ourselves. Once we accept this truth, it will be easier to get over our heartaches and hardships and fly toward wholeness.

Moving on requires us to be accountable for our actions and responsible for our own happiness. No longer can anyone make us do something we don't want to do. Taking charge of our future involves making a life-changing shift from being chickens to being geese.

Imagine humanity becoming like geese and flying uniformly in a "V" formation. Together we would share a common vision and sense of community. Followers would encourage leaders by honking and cheering. Hip, hip hooray, geese lead the way!

When we wake up on the sunny side of the street and behave like geese, we will role model noteworthy attitudes and positive behaviors for the rest of the flock. One by one may we become like geese and soar together with hopes of making our world a better place.

Geese vs. Chickens

GEESE	CHICKENS
Do it	Talk about it
Make time	Waste time
See opportunities	See only problems
Notice what's right	Notice what's wrong
Find a better way	Don't want to change
Solve problems	Cause heartaches
Are part of the solution	Stay stuck in the problem

Respond	React
Expect success	Expect failure
Expect to pay the price	Have a sense of entitlement
Work hard	Hardly work
Listen to others	Talk excessively
Learn from others	Think they know it all
Look after one another	Are self-centered
Gather facts	Have opinions
Evaluate results	Assume outcomes
Celebrate	Pout

As you go through life from this day forward, ask yourself, "Am I acting like a goose or a chicken?" If you are not sure about your behavior, ask members of your Breakfast Club!

4

Confrontation Over Easy

LIFE IS HARD. No one said it would be easy. There will be stressful times, misunderstandings, confusion, tension, unmet expectations, and strained interactions with others. At times, we need to be assertive and confront others. The question is: will the confrontation be easy or hard, effective or ineffective? You will gain more respect and trust if you practice the art of *gentle* confrontation. Weekly dialogue at the Breakfast Club helps prepare us to communicate over easy with the "real" world.

The key word in confrontation is "easy." Take it easy. When confronting family members, friends, or co-workers about a difficult topic, remember that people often respond to the messenger more than the words themselves. The receiver begins to process information before we even say a word.

What does your body language say when you are confronting someone? Notice your posture, eye contact, facial expression, hand gestures, and personal presence. No one wants to be blown out of the water when they are being confronted. Take it easy and try to maintain a sense of openness and sincerity when giving feedback. Examples of gentle body language are relaxed facial features, using a soft, soothing tone of voice, making eye contact, open palms, and keeping your hands at your side. Examples of harsh body language are raising your voice, pursing your lips, pointing your finger at the other person, folding your arms across your chest, staring intensely, and pacing back and forth. Body language plays a huge role in the art of gentle confrontation.

The purpose of confrontation is not to get something off your chest in order to feel immediate relief. It means waiting for the right time and place to share feelings and thoughts with the other person. It is lovingly and gently telling the person what they need to hear, not what they want to hear. Effective outcomes using over easy confrontation require time, patience, and practice. You will become graciously assertive the more you practice the art of gentle confrontation on your way to building better boundaries.

5

Hard Boiled Boundaries

ASSERTIVE COMMUNICATION AND emotionally honest living require setting boundaries in order to promote balance, protect self, and preserve relationships. Healthy boundaries are defined and refined on the sunny side of the street.

What is a boundary you ask? A boundary is a line one draws to protect all or part of one's self from being manipulated, controlled, misunderstood, discounted, abused or wrongly judged. For example: Being asked by a neighbor once in a while to pick up their child from school and take her home is fine. Being expected to pick up their child every day with little thanks and no reciprocation is overstepping a boundary.

Boundaries promote safety, well-being, inner peace, positive relationships, health and happiness. Boundaries bring a sense of order to life and work. When we choose ownership of our life, our boundaries will define our identity. Healthy boundaries will attract respectful and healthy relationships.

The good news is most people will adjust to your boundaries; however, expect your boundaries to be challenged. It is important to know that people with unclear boundaries will have difficulty respecting yours.

The more you practice boundary setting, the greater sense of control you will feel over your life. Boundaries open the door to more effective communication and loving service. The outcome of consistent self-assured living is less time repairing broken hearts and more time enhancing your life and the life of others. You may even discover that boundary setting is the most freeing skill you have ever learned!

The Breakfast Club had eggs over easy this morning and we celebrated our steady progress towards health and happiness thanks to building better boundaries. Here are a few tips to help you set effective boundaries in your own relationships.

Building Better Boundaries

- Identify and claim your personal morals and beliefs
- Adhere to your profession's "code of ethics" and code of conduct

- Observe your body language and notice other people's body language
- Pay attention to your senses
- Listen to your intuition
- Allow the Holy Spirit to direct your actions
- Let your conscience be your guide
- Honor your feelings
- Pay attention when your soul lets you know you have been threatened, discounted, diminished, disheartened, shamed or hurt
- Ask for feedback from safe, trusting people regarding your boundaries and behavior
- Lessons repeat themselves in order for us to learn what we need to learn on a deeper level
- Fear is sometimes associated with boundary setting. Feel the fear and do it anyway!
- Facing and overcoming boundary challenges will help increase your self esteem
- Practice improves boundaries. Practice, practice, practice!
- Set clear agreements with others
- Uphold your commitments and promises
- Notice and observe people who say **"yes"** and **"no"** confidently
- Speak up! Say **"no"** when you mean no and **"yes"** when you mean yes
- Draw the line between you and boundary violators
- Stop and redirect the encounter whenever you feel controlled, manipulated or discounted. Withdraw

from the person or situation so you can step back, reflect, and appropriately respond to the circumstances
- Seek help from licensed, reputable professionals when guidance and therapy are needed
- Role model healthy boundaries until they become a daily habit. Keep in mind that boundaries have the potential to generate a life "over easy."

6

Eggstra Ha-Ha-Ho-Ho-He-He

WHY LAUGH? WHY not laugh? Some experts say laughter is the best medicine. Some patients say laughter is what helped them survive life threatening illnesses. Perhaps there is some truth to the notion that FUN is FUNdamental to wellness.

Think about the last time you had a hearty ha-ha-ho-ho-he-he laugh. I mean a good old belly laugh that made your entire body rock and roll. The kind of laughter that forced funny noises from your mouth and made you snort. The time you laughed so hard you had to bend over and hold your ribs while you wiped the tears from your eyes. When was the last time laughter made you feel this good?

I don't now about you, but I want to laugh my way to health and happiness. Exercising our funny bone on a regular basis has the potential to give us eggstra health benefits by revitalizing our body from head to toe. If ha-ha-ho-ho-he-he laughter has the ability to revive the blood, energize the brain, stimulate the heart, expand the lungs, improve the immune system, and relax our nerves, sign me up for a free lifetime membership!

Speaking of membership, the Breakfast Club decided to meet monthly instead of weekly. We will begin measuring our ability to maintain positive change without weekly reinforcement. Ho Ho hope the Breakfast Club remains our sacred place for sustaining health and happiness. We've learned to laugh at ourselves and discover how humor enhances our relationship with others. Laughter occurs naturally at our Breakfast Club and we enjoy the benefits of living on the funny side of the street.

Scientists and healthcare professionals have been vigorously trying to prove the positive physical and psychological effects of laughter for the past three decades. Unfortunately the pharmaceutical drug companies aren't knocking down their doors to support this vital research. I think they spend a great deal of money on commercials listing possible side effects of their latest medications. Did you know that laughter does not need a prescription and doesn't have any side effects? Laughter at just the right moment helps the medicine go down. Holistic doctors and nurses recognize that compassionate laughter is a beneficial compliment to traditional medical treatments. Laughter is an old fashioned remedy that gives us hope and helps us cope.

If you want to learn more about therapeutic humor,

check out the Association for Applied and Therapeutic Humor's website: www.aath.org. In addition to the latest scientific research on humor and laughter, AATH provides wonderful resources for humor enthusiasts, as well as a yearly humor conference. Earning continuing education credits has never been so much fun! Imagine gathering with like-minded individuals who laugh and learn together for three days. Participants return home renewed and refreshed with lots of ideas for incorporating healthy humor into their lives.

The Breakfast Club is already signed up for next year's AATH humor conference. In the meantime, stay tuned for healthcare studies that validate how laughter increases production of endorphins, T-cells, and histamines in addition to decreasing physical pain, muscle tension, depression and blood pressure. While the world is waiting for more good news, be sure to get your daily dose of humor so you don't miss out on the positive benefits of hearty ha-ha-ho-ho-he-he laughter.

Throughout my psychiatric nursing career, many people asked me for advice on humor and healing. In 1998 I nicknamed myself Nurse FUNshine and shared my sunny way of looking at life with anyone who would listen. I tried to role model healthy humor in the work place, as well as promote self care for nurses and caregivers. For years, Nurse FUNshine presented workshops and programs on wellness, stress management, team building and humor. When participants left a conference and reported that they went home and incorporated healthy humor, laughter and fun into their homes, schools, churches, work places, and communities, it was affirmation that Nurse FUNshine's mission was being fulfilled. Quick wit, enthusiasm, audience participation and a cheerful spirit helped me become a sought after speaker.

Looking back, I believe it was Nurse FUNshine's "original" handouts filled with practical advice that accelerated my public speaking career. To honor sunny side up traditions, here are a few ha-ha-ho-ho-he-he tips from "Nurse FUNshine." May these FUN ideas and your very own Breakfast Club help "lighten up" your life.

Ha-Ha-Ho-Ho-He-He Humor Tips

1. Educate your family, friends, boss and co-workers about the benefits of healthy humor, then gain their support for the use of appropriate humor, play and FUN.
2. Create a colorful, cheerful, lighthearted, inviting atmosphere at work and at home.
3. Designate a bulletin board, mirror or refrigerator for comic strips, cartoons, jokes, funny pictures, reminder notes, etc.
4. Start a humor collection. Network with FUN, positive, playful people. Be open, ready and willing to experience surprises and spontaneous FUN.
5. Celebrate more than just birthdays and weddings. Throw parties just because! Incorporate the element of surprise into your daily activities.
6. Thank family, friends and coworkers with heart

warming gifts such as hand written notes, baked goods, warm fuzzies, balloons, flowers, etc.
7. Schedule joy breaks in your daily routine. Make time and take time for heart to heart FUN activities.
8. Decorate Life! Gather together for simple pleasures and FUN traditions during the holidays and summers. Take pictures so you and your loved ones can relive the memories and experience the joy over and over!
9. Get involved in the spirit of giving all year round. Practice random acts of kindness daily. Good deeds equal good karma. A smile on your face is a light to the world that says your heart is at home.
10. Sponsor FUN theme days to "lighten up" your working world. FUN ideas include: wacky hats, silly socks, ugly ties, tacky tourists, joke contests, talent shows, and holiday decorations.
11. Create a FUN committee at your school, place of work, organization, etc. The FUN committee will need administrative support and resources to plan and facilitate something FUN for the whole group at least 2 – 3 times per year.

As a result of these humor tips, many people reported that they successfully created a "lighter" home, work and/or school setting. Breakfast club members noted increased laughter and FUN in their personal and professional lives. I received valuable feedback indicating that willingness to live in the moment and the surrender of one's expectations helped discover or rediscover laughter and play. After years of teaching and preaching, I saw this FUN stuff change lives. The holes in peoples' souls began to fill up with joy. Restless hearts became content. Curiosity fueled my passion to promote healthy humor even more. Nurse FUNshine appeared in local newspapers and magazines to promote wellness workshops and help spread the good news about healthy humor.

Could the payoff for choosing to laugh be health and happiness? People stopped "doing" and started "being"; Clergy, healthcare workers, teachers, lay persons, cancer survivors, children, even morticians affirmed that Nurse FUNshine had been called to the "duty of delight" and my mission was to lead with laughter.

Heartfelt comic relief is more than just a joke or two. If laughter is going to change the world, the first lesson is the difference between healthy, compassionate humor and harmful, heartless humor. May compassionate ha-ha-ho-ho-he-he humor heal our bodies, minds and souls.

HEALTHY HUMOR	**HEARTLESS HUMOR**
Starts with a **smile**	Begins with **sarcasm**
Sparkles with a look of **love**	**Stings** with a **harsh** glance
Displays **kind, gentle** gestures	Makes **cruel** and **callous** remarks
Promotes **natural** laughter	Forces **fake** laughter
Bonds people together	**Divides** one another
Enhances self	**Defeats** others

Laughs at self and **with** others	Laughs only **at** others
Energizes the Soul	**Shames** one's spirit
Performs **considerate** deeds	Displays **insensitive** behavior
Promotes **teamwork**	Reinforces **self-centeredness**
Decreases tension	**Increases** tension
Produces **relaxation**	Creates **negative** stress and anxiety
Builds **confidence**	**Destroys** self worth
Involves and **embraces** others	**Manipulates** and **controls** others
Is **assertive** and **optimistic**	Becomes **aggressive** and **pessimistic**
Offers **hope** and helps us **cope**	Leaves behind **hurt** and **anger**
Creates contagious "**We**" go	Causes infectious **ego**

7

Don't Be a Chicken!

IF YOU ALWAYS do what you have always done, you will always be exactly where you already are. Do you often make statements such as these? *I like my life. I feel in control. I like my ducks to be in a row. My life is meticulously planned and predictable. I don't want to leave my comfort zone.*

Sounds boring. Why not dare to be different? Take some risks. Life is an adventure. Fasten your seatbelt and enjoy the ride! Once we view life as a journey, we learn to be grateful during the good times and graceful during the tough times. Learning to ride the waves of life becomes a daily challenge. Some days we will soar high on eagle's wings and other days we will hold on for dear life. The trick is to hang on and learn to ride the waves.

How we ride the waves is more important than how

long the waves last. Are you riding the waves in constant fear or are you riding the waves with faith, hope, and confidence? Children ride waves the best. They are risk takers filled with anticipation and excitement. Children's imaginations hitch their souls to the stars and protect their hearts from fear. Kids don't worry about how long the waves will last; they simply trust the process and enjoy each adventure. No wonder we love to spend time with children. Don't be a chicken ... let the child within you come out to play!

Adults need to set aside time to dream and play and laugh and love. Playing is the secret of youth. Take some risks and do something spontaneous. Play a game without rigid rules and strict score keeping. Play just for the fun of it. You will surprise others and maybe even surprise yourself. If nothing else, you will take a risk and experience something new and different. Taking a risk is kind of like taking a mini vacation from reality. Taking risks doesn't mean being careless and destructive with your life. Taking risks suggests doing something out of the ordinary from your everyday routine. Taking risks is about changing your mind on purpose, thinking outside the box, taking chances, riding the waves and chasing your dreams. Don't be a chicken ... try some of the following ideas and enjoy the ride of your life!

Don't be a Chicken ... Take Some Risks

- Take a new or different way to work once a week. Plan a few extra minutes so you can enjoy the

scenery along the way. Make a game of commuting and count how many different routes bring you to work. Who knows, this adventure may help you discover alternate routes in case of road closures or emergency evacuations.
- Stop and buy road side vegetables, fruit, honey, etc. You will appreciate eating fresh, local products, as well as meet interesting people outside your usual social circle. People + stories = adventures.
- The next time you go out to eat, choose a restaurant from an ethnic group other than your own. Different cultures cook with different herbs and spices. It is a culinary adventure to experience delicious food from other countries. Your taste buds will thank you! Be sure to ask questions like what does "hot" really mean and what are the most popular dishes you serve? Take advice from the regular patrons when choosing your main entree. Bon Appetite!
- Pull out those family recipes and cook books you collect. Find some favorite recipes, then plan and cook a meal from scratch. It is highly recommended to involve other family members in this cooking adventure.
- When traveling for work or pleasure and time allows, stop at antique stores, flea markets, garage sales, estate sales and going out of business sales. You might just find the perfect gift for the person who has everything or perhaps you will find the bargain of a lifetime. If nothing else, the browsing adventure is priceless!

- Save some extra money for a day of retail therapy. Take a day off work so you don't have to fight the Saturday crowds and go shopping somewhere other than your home town. Search the map for a city within 60 miles that is large enough to have a mall. If the city has a mall, they probably have a Marshall's, Ross, TJ Maxx, or Stein Mart. Invite one or two friends to come along for the fun.
- Here are a few tips to make your shopping trip a fun adventure. First, set a spending budget, take cash, and leave your credit cards at home. Next, agree to spend only 30 minutes in each store. Meet up front at the designated time and proceed to the next store. When undecided about a piece of clothing or household item, play the "how much would you pay for it" game before looking at the price tag. If it is that amount or lower, buy it. If the price is higher, put it back on the shelf or rack. You will be proud of your purchases and discover a whole new meaning for retail therapy. Power shopping usually ends with a home-cooked comfort meal from Cracker Barrel Country Store.
- **CAUTION MEN**: If your wife or girlfriend drags you along for a day of shopping, bring your favorite book or magazine and find a comfortable chair close to the dressing rooms. Better yet, agree to shop at places you like, as well as places your significant other likes. Think retail therapy for two!
- Welcome the new person in your apartment complex or the new family in your neighborhood. Take them

a modest welcome gift and home cooked meal. Offer them assistance in getting acquainted to the area and make them a list of reputable repair men and local businesses.
- Go somewhere different for your vacation this year. Perhaps there is a place you always wanted to visit ever since you saw it in one of those travel magazines or commercials. Maybe you want to revisit a place you went to when you were a little boy or girl. Since your family goes to the beach every summer, this summer you may want to go camping in the mountains. How about taking several day trips to interesting places near your home that you have never been to? Everyone should have the pleasure of staying in a cozy bed and breakfast once in his lifetime. Why not let the kids pick the vacation destination this year and next year the adults chose the destination? Vacation adventures are endless. There is something for everyone's budget, because it is the memories that make vacations special, not the destinations. Take a plane, train, bus, boat or automobile; just take a risk and visit some of the splendid places right here in America.
- Traveling is an adventure in itself. Airports, train depots, bus stations and highways are endless possibilities for fun times. Delays are inevitable, especially during the holidays. Be prepared and pack an extra set of clothes, toothbrush, snacks, a leisure book and travel games. Start having fun! You will

be surprised how many people want to join in the fun; all they need is permission.

One time we were delayed 8 hours in the Atlanta airport. We converted the waiting area into somewhat of a living room. We served snacks, played games, shared stories, laughed, turned strangers into friends, and made a lifetime of fond memories. Instead of complaining and dreading the delay, we turned our wait time into party time. What a FUN way to end our trip!

- When traveling, attend a local church service for a spiritual adventure. During the turning of the leaves one autumn, I attended a church in Massachusetts. It happened to be the weekend of their fall festival. What fun I had meeting these lovely folks, eating BBQ, playing games and winning one of the raffle prizes. There are endless surprise adventures waiting for curious visitors on the roads less traveled.
- Take a risk and let the people you love know it on a regular basis. Write a note and tell them how much you love them just because.
- Send a greeting card to a long distance friend or to someone who needs a little encouragement along life's road. Hand written words touch the heart and satisfy the soul.
- Initiate conversation before or after church with a total stranger. You may be surprised to learn that you both have something in common. Perhaps this person will become your new friend. Even better,

your warm welcome may be a much needed sign of hope and peace to a wandering visitor.
- After six to twelve months of risk taking, look back at all your adventures and reflect on how much your life has been enriched.
- Don't be a chicken! Pray for more serendipity and say "YES" to life!

8

A "Free-Range" Home

HOMEMADE, HOME GROWN, *home town, home for the holidays. There's no place like home. What home? Maybe I don't want to go home. Maybe I don't have a home. Someday I'm going to leave this place and start a home of my own.* Have you ever had these thoughts? The simple thought of *home* brings up a variety of mixed feelings, emotions and memories. Most homes consist of living quarters and testing grounds where family members learn to be a cohesive family. Home is a place where hens and roosters live together under one roof. We quickly learn our pecking order and carry out our inherited family roles to the best of our ability. A person's sense of self is initially shaped by one's caregivers and home life.

Within eighteen years or so, each child is shaped by

family, friends, neighbors, and community. Some grow up and never leave the nest. Some leave the nest early and never return. Some leave for awhile then return later in life. Our perceived image of home depends upon whether or not we lived in a free-range home or a home of bondage.

A home of bondage is like being in captivity where most family members are walking on egg shells. The mood of the home is dependent upon unpredictable parents or caregivers. The house rules are clear: don't laugh, don't cry, don't think for yourself. Tension fills the air most waking hours and survival skills for resilience are learned early in life.

A dysfunctional Breakfast Club usually surfaces which connects the family members in a twisted sort of way. A secret Breakfast Club may emerge to maintain a sense of control and keep a select group of family members sane. A home of bondage evokes emotional intuitiveness and flexibility which will prove to be very beneficial as offspring leave home and journey through life. Back at the house of blues, everyone seems sad and unhappy; yet no one will leave the nest and "free" himself due to a tremendous fear of failure. Eventually the hens and roosters escape the nest one way or another and search for an alternative home on the range. They are "free" at last.

A free-range home is a heartwarming place. It feels safe, comfortable, and nurturing. Some say a happy home is a sacred place. It's where people are "free" to be themselves without judgment or ridicule. A free-range home is where you learn the value of hard work, honest living, respect, and perseverance. Home life teaches you to rely upon God, each other and to believe in yourself.

Breakfast clubs happen on a regular basis because conversation, sharing, dreaming and encouragement are the main courses. "Free" thinking creates independence and self confidence. Friction is normal and expected, yet disagreements and conflicts are handled with satisfactory outcomes. Discipline, love, compromise and forgiveness set us "free" to return to our true selves. Our home team becomes our support team, as we help one another accomplish goals, overcome heart aches and live a "free" life. Home is where we learn to fill our time and space. Home is where we are taught the difference between being alone and being lonely. Home is where we study the meaning of love. We take our positive childhood experiences with us and spend our adult lives creating our own Breakfast Clubs and free-range homes.

The type of home we create depends upon a variety of influences. Many hens and roosters move on and establish satisfying home lives. It doesn't matter whether we come from a free-range home or a home of bondage; what matters is that we have a genuine desire to establish the kind of life every human being deserves. Valuable childhood lessons along with creative thinking and acquired knowledge help build a magnificent home on the range.

The free-range home we create is inviting and warm. Company is welcome and encouraged. Family and friends gather back home because they want to, not because they feel obligated. We begin our own Breakfast Clubs. Family traditions live on. Life is good. Life is full. Living in a free-range home is definitely home sweet home.

Suggestions for Creating a "Free-Range" Home

- Don't worry about what the neighbors have and don't have. Appreciate and be content with what you have.
- Live comfortably, yet beneath your means
- Schedule social gatherings, welcome spontaneous get togethers, and allow ample quiet time for individual reflection and renewal
- Set up an informal gathering area within your home where family and friends can relax and visit without distractions
- Turn off the TV unless you or your family members are watching a specific show, movie, or sporting event. Limit the time you spend watching TV and reading "bad" news
- Eat meals at the kitchen table, counter bar, or dining room table, not in front of the TV
- Play board games, card games and interactive games. Assign one night a week or one night a month as family game night. If space allows, have a table readily available for games and puzzles.
- Designate a quiet, well lit area for a reading nook
- Expect and plan for spur-of-the-moment company
- Make and freeze or buy several appetizers. Heat them up when you have guests. You will actually

have time to enjoy their company instead of spending all your time in the kitchen.
- Choose comfortable chairs for your dining room and kitchen tables
- Use that special china and silver for more than just holidays
- Allow enough time at sit down meals for casual conversation
- Listen more, talk less. Give advice only when specifically asked.
- Find things to laugh about
- Create a home where family and friends feel safe to laugh and cry
- Remember that everyone who passes through your door brings you happiness…some when they enter, some when they leave!

9

Baby Chicks ... Tickle Them, Please!

OLD MCDONALD HAD a farm, ee ii ee ii oo. We don't need a farm to raise baby chicks, but we do need some guidance with this parenting stuff. Instead of financing offspring, parents need to spend meaningful time raising their children. There is a difference between buying their love and winning their hearts. Sometimes the differences appear early in life. Other times power struggles surface during adolescence and create a testing ground for limit setting. Life on earth passes quickly and baby chicks grow up to become young men and women right before our very eyes. The stages from infancy to teenager seem like yesterday. Where did all the time go?

Take time to nurture your children. Kids want, need, and crave attention. They want your full attention, not just a superficial "uh huh" or "wait a minute." Put down that cell phone, get off that computer, quit watching drama TV, and spend some quality time with your children. One way or another, children will get your attention through positive or negative behaviors. Spending valuable time with your children is an investment that pays off sooner or later.

Several times the Breakfast Club invited our children to our gathering and my oh my did we have a memorable time! Children are authentically open, honest and playful. Kids don't remember how many minutes or hours you spend with them; kids remember the time you spend with them doing worthwhile activities. When was the last time you did something totally for fun with your children? You probably laughed and acted silly. Remember the look on their faces and the light in their eyes? You tickled their souls and guess what? Tomorrow they want to be tickled again.

That's right, tickle those baby chicks. Laugh and children laugh with you. Laughter is a heartfelt activity that tickles the soul. When we are genuinely interacting with children, we experience a state of joy about "being" instead of "doing." Most kids are naturally joyful. Seems like it's the grown ups who need permission to laugh and play. When we relax and become a part of our children's world, something magical happens. Laughing and playing with children breaks down our protective walls and prevents our hearts from hardening. That's because laughter is a gift that keeps on giving. Humor has the ability to strengthen relationships and promote healing, so open your heart and tickle your baby chicks!

There is a time to laugh and a time to weep. A time to reward and a time to discipline. Our role as caregivers is to be the parents, not our children's friends. Children and adolescents need love and discipline. Tough love is a necessary ingredient for healthy growth and development on the sunny side of the street. Parents who take responsibility and set up family guidelines, rules and expectations bestow their children a better chance towards health and happiness. If there are two parents in the household, they both need to agree and wholeheartedly support these standards. Children are clever. They will recognize the weak link and go ask the other parent for a denied request. Undermining the parent's authority becomes like a well played game of chess.

Parents need to be compassionate, cautious, caring, consistent and careful. If your children live in more than one home, it is crucial that both parents try to comprise for the children's sake regarding rules and structure. Do the best you can do with the limited amount of time you have with your children. Let your kids know that you love them and you are trying to be a decent parent. Be sure household guidelines and rewards are clear and known to everyone involved in child rearing. Explain how you as parents will help them achieve these family values. Once the family foundation is in place, it is up to the children to live accordingly or pay the consequences. Some days you will tickle and hug them. Other days you will discipline them and redirect their behavior.

Parents don't need to show their children who's the boss; they already know. However, there will be times when they test the limits to find out who is really in charge. Always remember to stay in control of your own feelings and behavior when disciplining your children.

Parents need to role model healthy behavior as you help shape your children's behavior. Consequences should teach not punish. When consequences correspond with the undesirable behaviors, children are presented the best opportunities for positive change. Shaping children's behavior is about choices, not control. Some behaviors require limit setting; other behaviors mandate immediate action. The more we practice effective parenting skills, the less time we spend yelling, crying and picking up the pieces of broken hearts. When parents don't allow children to experience consequences, we are really hurting them more than we are helping them. By the way, when kids are naughty wait until later to tickle them!

A Sunny Side Approach to Setting Limits

1. Identify the unacceptable behavior (focus on the behavior not the child)
2. Explain why the behavior will not be tolerated
3. Offer your child a positive option followed by a negative consequence

4. Allow time for his decision
5. Acknowledge and affirm good choices or carry out consequence
6. View decision making as a lesson in choices, not disappointments in life

Parenting is loads of hard work, a lot of prayers and a little bit of luck. The Breakfast Club came in handy many times throughout the child rearing years. Occasionally the Breakfast Club called an emergency meeting to help one of our members in a parenting dilemma. We parents stick together like birds of a feather! Some phases in child rearing are patiently tolerated, but most chapters in parenting are thoroughly enjoyed! Family traditions and rituals may seem corny, but festive activities keep us grounded and help us celebrate important milestones in life. It is a given that parents will make mistakes, but the good times outweigh the bad times. Children teach parents the value of unconditional love while parents instill the love of learning in kids. Why not view your child-raising years as an investment towards the future? May children grow up to become fine young adults who are responsible citizens and give back to their community. Hmmm I wonder if our children will take care of us when we are too old to tickle ourselves.

Parenting Pointers

- Name and claim your current parenting style
- Capitalize and utilize your parenting strengths

- Identify areas needing improvement and work towards positive change
- Practice parenting skills, review outcomes, revise behaviors, repeat
- Spend more time observing, noticing, and affirming your children
- Spend less time dictating, demanding and controlling your children
- Talk to your children, not at them
- Don't micromanage your children's daily lives
- Choose your battles wisely. Save your parental power for the BIG issues
- Don't waste your time and energy arguing with your children
- Instill a love of learning within your child, not just memorization
- RELAX ... toddlers and pre-schoolers learn through playing
- Cuddle and hold your baby often. Gently rub his head, back and feet
- Tickle, giggle, laugh, play, repeat
- Read books to your children. Visit the library and book stores often
- The family that prays together, stays together
- Strive towards joyful obedience as your family's spiritual goal
- Take your children to church regularly
- Limit and monitor TV time, video/Nintendo time, cell phone use and internet time
- Children need fresh air, regular physical activity,

plenty of pure water, nutritious meals and healthy snacks. Make wellness and fitness fun.
- Designate homework time and space so it becomes a week day routine
- Help children with homework, but don't do homework for them
- Back off when you find yourself working harder and want a desired change more than your children do. Remember and remind yourself that discomfort motivates positive change. If you do things for your children, they will not feel the pressure nor learn their intended lesson.
- Reward good grades. Raise the standards when your children are bored or settling for average, yet have the capabilities to do better.
- If your child is not capable of making A's, don't expect and demand A's. B's are above average and C's are average. Kids cannot do all things perfectly, especially when they are active in sports and hobbies.
- Encourage your children to be a part of something and do it well instead of being a part of everything and feeling like they are not good enough.
- Well rounded children seem better adjusted and more content than perfectionist, moody, uptight kids
- Make your home a gathering place. You will get to know your children's friends, as well as create a safe haven for "hanging out."
- Throw an annual party of some kind. (Back to School, Halloween, Valentines, Easter, Summertime, etc.) Make it a yearly tradition. Kids love to play games and act silly up to about the 5th or 6th grade.

- Set a curfew starting in Jr. High. As your children become older, raise or lower the curfew depending on how responsible they act.
- Parents usually think their children are better athletes, musicians, students, etc. than they really are. It's hard to be objective when you are emotionally attached to the situation. Be careful what you say in front of your children about their coaches and teachers. They will carry your attitude onto the field, and/or into the classroom.
- Instead of parents getting over involved with coaches' or teachers' decisions, simply encourage your children to meet with their coaches/teachers and find out what they can do differently or better to get more playing time or better grades. Have your children share this information with you during a dinnertime conversation. Encourage children to set their own goals for improvement and identify ways they can visually and objectively measure their own progress.
- Make an effort to be a "safe" and predictable parent. Children have a tendency to share more good news and bad news with parents who are calm, cool, level-headed and don't over react.
- Start a Breakfast Club for parents. Help yourself while you help other parents become effective, loving, responsible and FUN parents.
- Encourage your children to go away for educational adventures, summer camps, mission trip experiences and college. The more they travel and see how the rest of the world lives, the better "home" appears.

- Cherish every moment you have with your children. Whether they are 3 months old, 3 years old, 13 years old, or 30 years old, enjoy every minute you spend making memories with your children.
- Take plenty of pictures along the way. Reliving sunny side up memories will tickle your heart and soul for a lifetime!

10

Cracking Up

JUST ABOUT EVERY adult has watched "One Flew Over the Cuckoo's Nest." We either love that movie or hate it. The unsettling reality is that most people see themselves or their family members in the characters. We smile and tell ourselves that the characters really remind us of our in-laws. Wink, wink!

The truth of the matter is that cracking up is not all that bad. Cracking up pushes us to the edge, but rarely do we go over the edge. Instead, we hang on to hope and learn valuable lessons up close and personal. Hard times test our character and faith. We dig down deep and find amazing survival strength we didn't know we possessed. We fall on our knees, ask God to help us make it through the night, and promise to walk a straighter path. The dark night of our soul becomes a major wake-up call towards an authentic life centered around love. Breakfast Clubs are often discovered in the midst of emotional pain and cracking-up as a means of carrying us beyond the dark side of the moon. Snap, crackle, pop!

Shake, rattle and roll is a mild form of cracking up. Many people experience this phenomenon on a regular basis. It's when something or someone grabs a hold of our psyche and we perceive life differently from that awakening point. We learn a valuable lesson from the experience and adjust our attitude accordingly. Life goes on and we become skilled at responding to shake, rattle and roll occurrences. We change; we grow; we persevere.

The sooner we respond to shake, rattle and roll events, the better equipped we become in honoring our feelings, choosing happiness, dealing with heartaches, and preventing disasters. Effective coping skills learned from shake, rattle and roll situations help protect us from cracking up.

I experienced a shake, rattle, and roll situation in 2009 when my adult triathlete son suddenly lost vision in his left eye. At first the four of us shook with fear. Within a few days we pulled together like an amazing team and rattled every connection we had to seek the best medical care possible. We rolled with the diagnosis and hoped for the best. Thankfully my son's eyesight returned and he continues to compete in IronMan competitions. This up close and personal shake, rattle and roll experience taught our family how to persevere in the midst of unimaginable circumstances and serve one another with love.

Meltdowns are considered a moderate form of cracking-up. Meltdowns are characterized by intense feelings, volatile emotions, gut wrenching pain, and acute awareness about one's self and/or situation. We may temporarily lose control but are usually jolted back to reality with enhanced clarity and newly acquired knowledge. A deeper understanding of personal power emerges and acceptance becomes our middle name. We are changed from the inside out and there is no going back.

The lessons from meltdowns are more than "ah ha" moments; they can be compared to lightening bolts of spiritual transformation and divine intervention. We regroup, refocus and recover. Sometimes we can't believe how foolish we've been. Sometimes we question why we didn't see it coming. Other times we admit our shortcomings and make amends. How or why meltdowns happen doesn't matter. What matters is that we had an epiphany and now life makes sense. Common sense prompts us to shake, rattle and roll a little more often so we don't have to experience as many full blown meltdowns.

I experienced my own meltdown recently. My book completion deadline was extended for the 5th time; my son's black lab disappeared; my daughter got a speeding ticket; my husband caught the flu, and then poof! It was my turn to be sick. As I allowed myself to lie in bed for one full day, people contacted me with requests for my time, talent, advice, and assistance. Since I wasn't feeling like my usual cheerful self, I said "no thank-you" to everyone's requests. What a relief! Feeling "bad" wasn't so "bad" after all. I managed to rest, reflect, and recommit to finishing this book by my 53rd birthday. A clearer perspective of my own wants and needs became evident in less than 24 hours. A record miracle meltdown recovery and personal victory!

I must confess, I was ready to end this chapter on a serious note and write some valuable information about mental illness. About half way through the week, God decided to teach me a few more things about meltdowns. Whoever says God doesn't have a sense of humor must not have any sense at all!

I was preparing for two speaking engagements, getting both of our family businesses' tax information together for the CPA and working on sales tax that is due by the 20th. In addition, I was completing my daily tasks that are more than enough work for two full-time employees. Once again I found myself playing the role of wonder woman. It's been such a long time I thought, let me run with it and see how much I can accomplish in the next three days.

Some of you know the wonder woman/superman drill. Day one felt great. I was on top of the world. The "high" of accomplishing my short-term goals gave me more energy than I had in weeks. Day two should have been my wake up call, a jolt back to reality, awareness and insight that something had to give. But no! I'm stubborn so I buckled down and persevered. I worked through lunch while everyone else took lunch and stayed late when everyone else went home at 5:00 pm. Anxiety, anger and resentment attacked me like a thief in the night. Right before my very eyes, I turned into a fighting rooster. I was wound up tight and I desperately needed to pick a fight with someone, anyone, probably the next person I met.

I managed to be nice to my husband that evening and went to bed early to keep myself out of hot water. Lo and behold the CPA arrived the next day for our 3:00 pm appointment and asked me how I was doing. A loaded question since I was overwhelmed and at the verge of another meltdown. At first I gave the usual "fine" response, and then little by little, I unloaded about everything and everyone who was contributing to my current state of overwhelming stress. The CPA crossed his arms and gave me a serious look as he said, "sounds like you need some help."

I laughed out loud. His look intensified. I laughed again nervously then got a grip and regained my composure. Instantly I realized that the CPA meant help with our family business and office. I thought he meant help in giving up my role as wonder woman.

I smiled wholeheartedly, took a deep breath, felt the sting of embarrassment and quickly gathered my thoughts and emotions. I humbly thanked him for his feedback and sat back in my chair contemplating the CPA's words. His crucial message punctured my grandeur behavior and caused a major gut reaction about choices within my soul. I was grateful that another professional did a mini Breakfast Club intervention on the spot and candidly gave me permission to get help. Sometimes we need permission to step out of our role as wonder woman and super man. Asking for and accepting help is just what Nurse FUNshine needed for preventing future meltdowns. Just say "YES" to help! From shake, rattle and roll to profound meltdowns, we become stronger, wiser and more resilient.

The third type of cracking-up is a severe and serious brain disorder that requires professional help; yet very few people want to talk about it. Mental illness affects millions of people, yet most people know very little about mental illness. It is acceptable to have diabetes or heart disease in our society, but unfortunately there remains much stigma to overcome regarding mental illness.

Mental illness is not due to personal weakness, lack of character, or not enough willpower. It is an illness that disrupts a person's thinking, feelings, mood, behavior and body. What the world needs to know is that mental illness is treatable. With proper therapy, counseling, medication, self help groups, Breakfast Clubs and other community services, most people with mental illness get well and lead productive, content lives.

The first step is seeking help. Sometimes a person knows he needs help and other times it is loved ones who intervene and make the difficult decision to seek professional help. Successful outcomes require an accurate diagnosis, individualized treatment plan, fine tuned medication management and patient compliance. Whether the mental illness is depression, bipolar disorder, anxiety disorder, schizoaffective disorder, paranoid schizophrenia, or an eating disorder, taking steps towards recovery are essential factors in the treatment of mental illness. For more information contact your local community mental health center and/or the National Alliance on Mental Illness (N.A.M.I.) at www.nami.org or 1-800-950-6264.

It is very important to know that urgent help is necessary when a person becomes suicidal, homicidal, a danger to self or others, gravely disabled, and/or acutely psychotic/bizarre. If your family member or loved one is experiencing these signs and symptoms, contact your local mental health hospital or emergency room for <u>immediate</u> help, assessment and treatment.

11

Empty Nesters ... YES!

TIME FLIES BY. Before we know it, babies turn into toddlers and toddlers grow up to be children. Children become adolescents who develop into young adults and leave the nest. My oh my how time flies by on the sunny side of the street. Hopefully young adults are prepared, equipped, and excited to leave the nest.

Mom and Dad are excited and ready for their departure. Or are they? The reality of an empty nest hits some couples like a ton of bricks. The big day comes and the last offspring leaves the nest for college, the military, or a full-time job. Parents hold back their tears, hug them goodbye and send them off to build a nest of their own.

A week or two flies by; ok time drags by. The house is quieter than usual because some of the laughter has disappeared. The empty places at the dinner table are constant reminders that children are missing from the nest. For weeks we struggle to look on the bright side of our parental freedom. The bathroom stays clean for an entire week; the grocery bills are lower, laundry is a cinch and we can watch whatever we want on TV. But if this is life on the sunny side of the street, where's the joy? Could the thrill be gone? We parents look at each other and ask, "What's wrong with us?" We need to get a grip!

For some couples, the empty nest becomes a trying time of endurance and survival. If the only thing parents truly have in common is their children, the empty nest era will become a huge challenge in the marriage. After much soul searching, some couples rekindle their love for one another and build a stronger foundation for the long run.

Other couples, however, wait patiently for their empty nest to arrive and acknowledge the truth about their unhappiness. Now that the children are gone, the couple gives each other permission to take off separately on their own paths of freedom. Both husband and wife knew for years that they were drifting apart and neither one wanted to invest anymore time and energy into their marital relationship. No Breakfast Club can help save the marriage. The combination of an empty life plus an empty nest creates independence. Two different kinds of empty nesting, but both couples are finally free!

Many couples experience the freedom of the empty nest like a breath of fresh air. Every long distance telephone conversation is affirmation that baby chicks are adjusting well to their new adult life away from home.

This anticipated milestone is what we longed for since high school. Our children are finally on their own journey towards independence, health, happiness and success. We are happy and proud parents. Let freedom ring!

We still have plenty of time to enjoy life and are healthy enough to travel. In addition, we still love and respect each other, as well as value each other's company. YES, we finally arrived at the door of our very own empty nest. All we need is a little attitude adjustment to spice up our life!

Some couples are fast learners when it comes to parental freedom. It doesn't take long for them to reconnect with old friends. Imagine going out for dinner at the spur of the moment and taking spontaneous weekend trips to local bed and breakfasts. Some couples discover a love for fine wine, good food, fellowship, and regular social gatherings. Besides daily work routines, empty nesters can do what they want, when they want, how they want. The pressure of school activities, commitments, and schedules disappear like the wind.

For these empty nesters, life becomes a zealous and fulfilling ride. Spontaneous romance returns. In the evenings there is plenty of time to share thoughts, blessings and dreams. Laughter resurfaces and there appears to be plenty of situations to laugh about. T.V. is an option, but most nights are filled with reading books and intimate conversations. Empty nesters can even go to bed early just because they wish! Reconnecting as husband and wife is exciting, plus there is nothing like a break from kids before becoming grandparents. A note of caution: take advantage of the empty nest while you can.

Adult children sometimes return to the nest, for additional financial and emotional support. Resist this urge if at all possible. For one couple I know, their short-lived empty nest now hosts three generations under one roof. They went from an empty nest to a full house. Perhaps this is a temporary assignment of love and loyalty; besides, what parent wouldn't open the door and welcome his children back home?

Invite them in, but remember, your adult children and grandchildren are visitors in your home. Please don't convert your well deserved empty nest into a cozy retreat for them. The goal is to give them a helping hand until they are back on their feet and can once again leave the nest. Think of your home as their temporary nesting place, not a permanent comfort zone. Say hello. Set a time frame for departure. Say good-bye and enjoy your empty nest!

12

Roosters Rule the World with Wisdom

HATS OFF TO the older generation. Your wisdom guides the world. May your golden years be filled with sunshine, laughter and fond memories.

Seniors know that wisdom is more than just knowledge; it's experience, insight, plus good judgment that lead to brain power. The older generation passionately and bravely fought for our country's freedom and whole heartedly believes "The Pledge of Allegiance" is an oath to the United States of America. We are one nation, under God, indivisible, with liberty and justice for all. Thank you, senior citizens, for your wisdom, guidance and courage. May we carry on the family traditions, Breakfast Clubs and sacred rituals you taught us with dignity, honor and respect. May we acknowledge and understand that it takes mature roosters to rule the world with wisdom.

The younger generation is slowly realizing how much hard work and how many sacrifices were made by the older generation in order to make our world a better place. Seniors possess valuable knowledge and experience about the ups and downs of life. The wiser, older generation has been there and done that. They are ready, able and willing to share their wisdom with the younger generation. The older generation has valuable advice to pass on, stories to share and jokes to tell. Gathering regularly for a meal and conversation is a great way to start a Breakfast Club with older friends and relatives. Set aside some time to spend with senior citizens and listen to their stories. Relax, pull up a chair and sit awhile, Grandma and Grandpa are going to share their secrets to a long and happy life on the sunny side of the street. Long live Breakfast Clubs.

Rules for a Long and Happy Life

1. Fresh air, flowers and sunshine are good for the soul.
2. Read the Bible. Communicate with God daily through prayer and songs. One day you will thank Grandma for dragging you to church.
3. Extend God's love to others. Spread goodwill throughout your home and community. When you have enough, be grateful. When you have more than enough, be generous.
4. Stretch your mind. Learning enhances creativity

and develops wisdom. An education offers the opportunity to use your brain instead of your back.
5. Work for the best and expect the best. One day you will reap the benefits you deserve from all your hard work.
6. Spend your free time improving yourself so that you don't have time to criticize others.
7. Help others shine. Celebrate success, but don't get too big for your britches. Remember that teamwork is "we go" not "ego."
8. Take yourself "lightly" and your job seriously. Find things to laugh about everyday. Cherish your sense of humor.
9. Stand up and fight for what is right. Ask not what your community can do for you, but what you can do for your community.
10. Be proud of your heritage, yet respect the privilege that U.S. citizens are first and foremost Americans.
11. Let go of the past. Build a life filled with love, laughter, forgiveness and peace.
12. Know that you become like the company you keep.
13. Carry on family traditions and create some new ones along the way.
14. Appreciate and consume home grown, homemade, and whole grains because they complement healthy living.
15. Fill your grocery cart with mostly fresh food. When you can't get it fresh, buy frozen food. Sodium-laden canned goods should not be the staple of your diet.

16. The body craves and needs plenty of pure water daily. Soft drinks and sugary juices were meant to be occasional treats.
17. Read food labels. If you cannot pronounce the ingredients, don't buy the product. Stay away from high fructose corn syrup, artificial sweeteners, monosodium glutamate (MSG) and hydrogenated oils.
18. Stick with "real" butter, raw cane sugar, maple syrup, molasses, cold pressed olive oil, and locally grown honey. It is not worth saving a few calories to eat artificial coloring, chemicals and additives.
19. Buy organic produce and hormone free meats and dairy products from your local farmers' market or family farm co-op. Better yet, grow your own fruits and vegetables.
20. Ditch the "fad diet"; a sound mind plus clean eating along with an active lifestyle promotes health and happiness.
21. Happy is the person who has a B.M. every A.M.
22. Use natural soaps, lotions, shampoos and conditioners. Don't put anything on your body, skin, face or hair that you wouldn't put in your mouth.
23. Wash your clothes and dishes with natural detergents. Dishes and clothes are supposed to be clean and fresh not chemically treated.
24. Wash your hands regularly with natural soap and water to help prevent the spread of germs and disease. Always wash your hands before meals and after you use the restroom.

25. Get off that couch and move those muscles! Be thankful you don't have to walk several miles through rain or snow to go to school.
26. Never underestimate the power of good ole common sense.
27. When you fall down, and you will, get up, brush off the sting, stand tall, keep your chin up, regroup and march forward.
28. Join a Breakfast Club or start one of your own. Important characteristics of a healthy Breakfast Club include a structured group with a primary focus, guidelines, strict confidentiality, trust, punctuality, consistent attendance, active participation, emotional honesty, and an official opening and closing. Benefits from a healthy Breakfast Club include greater self awareness, improved confidence, better coping skills, a sense of belonging, enhanced health and genuine happiness.
29. When life gives you lemons, make lemonade.
30. Spend as much time as you can with the older generation. Cherish their wisdom and unconditional love. You will miss them when they're gone; however, your hearts will stay connected.
31. Look at the sunny side of everything.

Baker's Dozen

Living on the Sunny Side of the Street

TODAY IS THE final day of Breakfast Club 101 and the rest of our lives. Let's live life to the fullest. Merely existing is for the birds; we want to fly high "naturally" and land sunny side up. After weeks, months, or years, we eventually make it to the sunny side of the street. Our hearts have been changed from the inside out and our souls feel alive and well. We are eager to share our message of spiritual transformation and joyful living with others.

A few words of caution: easy does it. There will be times when we have to tone down our enthusiasm and joy. Our personal growth and prescription for happiness will not be applauded by everyone. We need to prepare ourselves for the fact that there will be family members and friends who will not be able to accept our genuine makeover and cheerfulness. The old saying that misery loves company is still true today. Love them anyway, but don't try to rescue and carry them to the sunny side of the street. Invite them to be a part of a Breakfast Club, but don't drag them along against their will. Meet them where they are and give them an opportunity to experience personal growth on their way to a better life. In the meantime fasten your seatbelt, secure your own oxygen mask, and offer hope to other Breakfast Club members.

There will be days when the sun doesn't shine on the sunny side of the street. Bad things happen to good people. When clouds blur our vision and we can't see clearly through our rose colored glasses, we need simple remedies to overcome the blues. Since pain, heartaches, and disappointments are part of life, why not be prepared? We can put gentle reminders and affirmations throughout our surroundings that encourage us to hang on for the ride. This too shall pass. Seek a Breakfast Club for advice and support.

Let's change our minds on purpose, fill our days with FUNshine and allow healing to take place. Put together a humor basket filled with riddles, magic tricks, silly gadgets, colorful stickers, child like band-aids, balloons, a slinky, silly putty, whistles, kazoos, comics, funny pictures, and clown noses. Share the humor basket with someone who needs a little tender loving care and miraculously notice how much better you feel! If you have a family member or friend in the hospital, bring him a humor basket. Creating a fun atmosphere will "lighten up" the environment and have a positive effect on almost everyone who enters his room. Sometimes laughter is the best medicine.

Another suggestion for overcoming gloom and doom is to develop a personal care plan with ideas that have potential to improve the quality of your life. Think Breakfast Club for one. Write your own customized action plan using tips and advice gathered from attending a variety of Breakfast Clubs. Create an individualized "Sunny Side Up" Prescription and add more FUNshine to your life. When you need to improve your attitude or mood, take out your "Sunny Side Up" Prescription and try one or more natural remedies. Make notes and evaluate the results from your positive actions. Add new ideas and activities to your "Sunny Side Up" Prescription. Refill often. Once you know what activities help cheer you up, you may not even need a list. Here is my cheerful prescription. Hope these ideas bring you a little FUNshine too.

Nurse FUNshine's "Sunny Side Up" Prescription

- Express yourself through music and movement. Dance like nobody's watching.
- Sing at church, sing in the shower, sing and connect with your soul
- Smile even if you have to fake it. There is a good chance that forcing a smile will eventually lead to a genuine smile.
- Follow a regular exercise regimen. Exercise is a

powerful antidote to a case of the blahs. Researchers say that rhythmic, continuous exercise such as dancing, jogging, bicycling, swimming and walking provide the widest range of psychological benefits.

- Reach out and give to others for a warm fuzzy feeling
- Take 3 - 5 slow, deep breaths. Breathe in through your nose, hold it for a few seconds, and then exhale through your mouth. Gently force out as much stale air as you can from your lungs.
- Create a joy list naming activities that you love to do. Take time weekly to do at least one thing from your joy list.
- Daydream for a temporary vacation from boredom.
- Go to a funny movie with someone who has a great sense of humor. Give each other permission to laugh out loud before you enter the theatre then laugh to your heart's content.
- Curl up on the couch or snuggle in bed and read an enjoyable book.
- Make bread. Using your hands to knead the dough and getting lost in an activity that absorbs your attention will help you relax.
- Enrich your daily routines. Turn cooking, flower arranging, cleaning and gardening into ordinary art.
- Treat your feet to a therapeutic foot bath. Soak both feet in a bucket or bowl filled with very warm (but not scalding) water for a few minutes. Transfer feet quickly to bucket or bowl with cold water for a few seconds. Return to the warm water and repeat process several times.

- Reward yourself for reaching fitness milestones, personal goals and professional accomplishments. Tangible rewards renew motivation.
- Keep a journal. Set aside 10 – 20 minutes regularly and write only for yourself. Journaling is an exercise in creative freedom. It will help you reflect, express, explore, problem solve and dream. People who journal regularly report increased awareness, clarity, empathy and happiness.
- Create a tea ritual. Take out your favorite tea cup. Boil or brew some water then pour into tea cup. Add herbal tea and steep for a few minutes. Place your hands around the warm tea cup. Smell the aroma as you slowly sip and enjoy your warm tea. Tea rituals are especially comforting on cold or rainy days.
- When all else fails, get a new hairstyle at the beauty salon, and let the "new" you emerge.

The world needs Breakfast Clubs now more than ever. The more time we spend living on the sunny side of the street, the less time we spend worrying about how long our serenity and happiness will last. Living one day at a time, we become fully present to each moment, yet anticipate and look forward to the future. We understand the difference between balance and boredom. We attempt to eliminate as much drama and chaos as possible from our lives. We respect ourselves and our decisions. We trust our thoughts, feelings and judgments. We do what we think is right. We become skilled at acceptance, tolerance, patience and willingness. We laugh more, cry more, love more and live more. We pay close attention to our hearts inner calling and recognize the need for regeneration of the human spirit. We accept the responsibility and take on the challenge to make a difference in our corner of the world. We let our light shine with hopes of healing our planet one person at a time.

Yes my friends, this sunny side up condition is contagious. Visualize wellness. Learn it, live it, pass it on. Ready or not, here comes the sun. Genuine health and happiness exists in a dozen combinations. Don't be a chicken… unscramble your life and act like a goose. Wake up, smell the coffee and start living on the sunny side of the street!